CANCER DIETS COOKBOOK FOR BEGINNERS

The complete cancer guide with super easy and tasty recipes

KATRINA THOMAS

TABLE OF CONTENTS

Introduction

Copyright©2023 By Katrina Thomas

Disclaimer

The information contained in this cookbook is not intended to replace professional medical advice. If you have any concerns about your health or nutrition, please consult with a qualified healthcare professional.

The recipes and information in this cookbook are intended to support a healthy lifestyle, but they are not a guarantee of health benefits or a substitute for professional medical treatment.

The publisher and authors do not assume any liability for any adverse effects that may result from the use of the information contained in this cookbook.

Introduction

Millions of individuals worldwide are impacted by the complex and deadly disease of cancer. Although there is no one specific cause of cancer, it is well known that lifestyle choices like nutrition can have a substantial impact on the onset and course of the illness.

The relationship between food and cancer has been the subject of extensive investigation in recent years, and mounting data point to the possibility that some diets may be protective against particular cancer forms.

With so many individuals turning to cancer-fighting diets in an effort to lower their risk of contracting the disease, the relationship between diet and cancer has become a hot topic in the world of health and wellness.

These diets frequently emphasize eating a lot of whole, unprocessed foods and limiting or avoiding foods like refined carbs, red and processed meats, and unhealthy fats that have been linked to an increased risk of developing cancer.

Cancer-Preventative Diets

There are numerous cancer-prevention diets, each with its own philosophy towards food and wellness. The following are some of the most well-known and investigated diets:

Diets that are mostly plant-based emphasize the consumption of a large variety of plant-based foods, such as fruits, vegetables, whole grains, legumes, and dairy, while restricting or avoiding animal products. It has been demonstrated that plant-based diets are protective against some cancers, particularly colorectal cancer.

Anti-inflammatory diets: Since inflammation plays a significant role in the onset and spread of cancer, many cancer-fighting diets put an emphasis on lowering it in the body.

While restricting or avoiding items that cause inflammation, such as sugar, processed carbs, and bad fats, anti-inflammatory diets often contain a high proportion of anti-inflammatory nutrients, such as omega-3-rich fish, leafy greens, and healthy fats.

The Mediterranean diet is an ancient dietary pattern that has been used for millennia in nations that border the Mediterranean Sea. It is characterized by a reduced intake of red and processed meats and a high intake of complete, unprocessed foods, such as fruits, vegetables, whole grains, nuts, and healthy fats.

Numerous cancers, including breast, colon, and prostate cancer, have been found to be protected against by the Mediterranean diet.

The ketogenic diet is a high-fat, low-carbohydrate diet that has become more and more well-known in recent years. It functions by causing the body to enter a state of ketosis, when it uses fat as fuel rather than carbohydrates.

Even though the ketogenic diet hasn't been thoroughly researched in relation to cancer, some evidence points to a potential therapeutic benefit for some cancers.

Juicing and smoothies are becoming more popular as ways to obtain a concentrated amount of nutrients in a manageable form. Consuming fruits and vegetables that are high in nutrients and low in sugar is a key component of cancer-fighting juice and smoothie diets.

Anti-inflammatory ingredients like turmeric, ginger, and chia seeds may also be added.

Each of these diets for combating cancer has its own approach to nutrition, and some might be better suited for particular people than others.

All cancer-fighting diets, however, emphasize eating whole, unprocessed foods and restricting or avoiding items that have been linked to an elevated risk of developing cancer.

Conclusion: While no single diet will guarantee immunity against cancer, there is mounting evidence that some cancer-fighting diets may help lower the risk of contracting the disease. Limiting or avoiding processed and harmful foods while increasing the consumption of whole, nutritious foods

CHAPTER 1

Overview of plant-based diets

A type of diet that focuses on consuming a lot of plant-based foods, like fruits, vegetables, legumes, and whole grains, while restricting or avoiding animal products is called a plant-based diet.

These eating plans are predicated on the notion that a diet high in unprocessed, whole foods from plants may act as a preventative measure against specific cancers.

The advantages of a plant-based diet

Reduced Cancer Risk: A substantial body of research points to the possibility that plant-based diets can lower the risk of certain cancers, particularly colon cancer.

Diets rich in fiber, antioxidants, and phytochemicals are thought to lower oxidative stress and inflammation in the body, which is thought to help prevent cancer.

Better Heart Health: Plant-based diets are low in saturated fat and cholesterol and high in nutrients that are good for the heart, like fiber, potassium, and magnesium.

It has been demonstrated that this vitamin combination lowers the risk of heart disease, the major cause of death worldwide.

Better Weight Management: Diets based on plants often contain few calories and a lot of fiber, which can help people feel fuller for longer and limit their food intake.

This may result in better weight management and a lower chance of obesity, which is known to increase the risk of developing cancer and other chronic diseases.

Better Gut Health: Plant-based diets are high in fiber, which is crucial for preserving a balanced gut microbiota. A balanced gut microbiota is linked to a lower risk of cancer and other chronic illnesses.

Environmental Sustainability: Diets based primarily on plants are more environmentally friendly than those including a lot of animal products.

Reducing our use of animal products can help lessen the negative effects our diets have on the environment because animal agriculture is a significant source of greenhouse gas emissions, deforestation, and other environmental issues.

Despite the fact that plant-based diets may have numerous health advantages, they can also lead to nutrient deficiencies, such as those in iron and vitamin B12, if not well planned.

To make sure that a plant-based diet is balanced and covers all of your nutritional needs, it is crucial to seek the advice of a healthcare professional or certified dietitian.

Plant Based Diet

1. Quinoa Bowl with Roasted Vegetables:

Ingredients:

1. Quinoa, one cup
2. 2 small sweet potatoes, cut into medium-sized chunks
3. a single huge red bell pepper, diced up.
4. 1 substantial zucchini, cut into small pieces.
5. 1 medium onion, peeled and cut into small pieces.
6. Olive oil, two tablespoons
7. pepper and salt as desired.
8. 1/4 cup feta cheese crumbles (optional)
9. herbs for garnish, fresh (optional)

Instructions:

1. Set the oven's temperature to 400°F (200°C).
2. Rinse the quinoa in a fine mesh sieve before adding it and 2 cups of water to a medium pot.
3. To cook the quinoa, bring the water to a boil, then lower the heat, cover the pan, and let the quinoa simmer for about 15 minutes, or until the water is absorbed.
4. Combine the finely diced sweet potatoes, red bell pepper, zucchini, and onion in a large mixing bowl.
5. Mix in the olive oil to evenly coat the vegetables.
6. Salt and pepper the vegetables before spreading them out on a sizable baking sheet.
7. The vegetables should be baked for 20 to 25 minutes, or until they are soft and just beginning to brown.
8. With the roasted vegetables added on top, serve the cooked quinoa in bowls.
9. If preferred, sprinkle with chopped fresh herbs and feta cheese.

2. Kale and lentil soup:

Ingredients:

1. 1 cup of green or brown lentils, washed in 4 cups of vegetable broth, along with 1 big onion, 2 cloves of minced garlic, 2 medium carrots, 2 stalks of celery, and 1 cup of chopped vegetables
2. 1 tomato diced can (14.5 oz)
3. 2 cups of chopped kale
4. pepper and salt as desired.
5. herbs for garnish, fresh (optional)

Instructions:

1. Heat a thin layer of oil in a big pot over medium heat. About 5 minutes after adding the onion, it should be tender.
2. Cook for a further five minutes after adding the minced garlic, diced carrots, and chopped celery to the saucepan.
3. Add the kale, diced tomatoes, vegetable broth, and rinsed lentils.
4. When the lentils are cooked, about 30 minutes after bringing the stew to a boil, turn the heat down and let it simmer.
5. To taste, add salt and pepper to the food. If preferred, top hot dishes with fresh herbs.

3. Ingredients for grilled portobello mushroom burgers:

1. I removed the stems from four huge Portobello mushroom caps.
2. Four whole-wheat buns
3. 4 cheese slices (optional)
4. Your choice of toppings, including lettuce, tomato, and other
5. Olive oil, two tablespoons
6. pepper and salt as desired.

Instructions:

1. Grill at a medium-high temperature.
2. Salt and pepper the Portobello mushroom tops after brushing them with olive oil.
3. The mushrooms should be grilled for four to five minutes on each side, or until soft and slightly browned.
4. The whole-grain buns should be lightly crisped after 2 minutes of grilling.
5. Put a grilled Portobello cap on the bottom of each bun before adding lettuce, tomato, cheese (if using), and any other desired toppings.

Overview of anti-inflammatory diets

Incorporating certain foods and avoiding others that are thought to increase inflammation in the body are the main goals of anti-inflammatory diets.

Inflammation is the body's normal response to injury, infection, or illness, but when it persists for an extended period of time, it can lead to the onset of many illnesses, such as cancer, heart disease, and autoimmune disorders.

The anti-inflammatory diet is based on the tenets of a Mediterranean-style diet, which places a strong emphasis on consuming a majority of plant-based foods, such as fruits and vegetables, whole grains, nuts, seeds, and legumes.

Additionally, it advises cutting back on your consumption of animal products, processed meals, and refined sugar while increasing your intake of beneficial fats like olive oil.

Advantages of An anti-inflammatory diet

- lowered risk of developing chronic diseases and improved general health
- better control of the symptoms of inflammatory diseases such as inflammatory bowel disease and arthritis
- Improved dietary control and maintenance
- improved blood sugar control and a decreased risk of type 2 diabetes
- cardiovascular disease risk reduction and improved heart health

Note: It's crucial to remember that while an anti-inflammatory diet may be advantageous for some individuals, it may not be suitable for all.

Anti-inflammatory diets

1. Avocado salsa and wild salmon:

1. 4 filets of wild salmon (6 ounces each)
2. To taste, add salt and pepper.
3. Olive oil, two tablespoons
4. To make the salsa:
5. 2 ripe avocados, chopped; 1 pint cherry tomatoes, quartered, and minced 1 jalapeno

6. two tablespoons of freshly chopped cilantro and one tablespoon of lime juice
7. To taste, add salt and pepper.

Instructions:
1. Set the oven to 400 °F. Use parchment paper to cover a baking sheet.
2. Olive oil should be brushed on after seasoning the salmon filets with salt and pepper.
3. On the prepared baking sheet, put the salmon filets and bake for 12 to 15 minutes, or until done.
4. In the meantime, mix the chopped avocado, cherry tomatoes, jalapenos, cilantro, lime juice, salt, and pepper in a medium bowl.
5. Serve the salmon filets topped with the salsa made from avocados.

2. Sweet potato and chickpea bowl with spices:
1. diced two medium sweet potatoes
2. 1 can of washed and drained chickpeas
3. Olive oil, two tablespoons
4. 1 teaspoon of cumin, ground
5. smoked paprika, 1 teaspoon
6. To taste, add salt and pepper.
7. Quinoa, one cup

8. 2-cups of water

9. Juiced lemon, half

10. 14 cups chopped fresh parsley

Instructions:

1. Set the oven to 400 °F. Use parchment paper to cover a baking sheet.

2. Combine the chopped sweet potatoes, chickpeas, cumin, paprika, salt, and pepper in a big bowl. When coated evenly, toss.

3. Bake for 25 to 30 minutes, or until the sweet potatoes are soft and the chickpeas are crispy, after spreading the mixture out on the prepared baking sheet.

4. Quinoa, water, and a dash of salt are combined in a medium pot in the meantime.

5. Boil, then turn down the heat and cover.

6. Cook the quinoa for 18 to 20 minutes, or until the water has been absorbed and the quinoa is soft.

7. Add the parsley and lemon juice and stir.

8. Along with the roasted sweet potato and chickpea mixture, serve the quinoa.

3. Stuffed bell peppers with turkey and spinach

1.   4 large, any color bell peppers
2.   1 pound of turkey, ground
3.   1 diced onion
4.   3 minced garlic cloves
5.   2 cups chopped fresh spinach
6.   1 diced tomato can
7.   one tablespoon dried basil
8.   To taste, add salt and pepper.
9.   1 cup of brown rice, cooked

Instructions:

1.   Turn on the 375°F oven.
2.   Line a baking pan with parchment paper.
3.   The bell peppers' tops should be cut off, and the seeds and membranes should be removed.
4.   Put the peppers in the baking pan that has been prepared.
5.   Cook the ground turkey in a sizable skillet over medium heat, breaking it up into small pieces as it cooks.
6.   When the onion is transparent, add it to the skillet along with the garlic.
7.   Add the diced tomatoes, chopped spinach, basil, salt, and pepper.
8.   Cook the spinach until it wilts.

9. Add the cooked rice and stir. Fill the bell peppers evenly with the mixture by spoon.

10. Bake the dish with the foil on top for 30–35 minutes, or until the filling is hot and the peppers are soft.

Overview of Mediterranean diet

The traditional foods of nations in the Mediterranean Sea region, like Greece, Italy, and Spain, are the foundation of the Mediterranean diet, which is an eating plan.

It is distinguished by a concentration on unprocessed, entire foods, such as:

I.   fruits and veggies in abundance

II.   Whole grains are used to make products like whole wheat bread and pasta.

III. legumes, such as beans and lentils, and nuts and seeds

IV.   is the main source of fat, olive oil

V.   modest consumption of fish and poultry

VI.   Consumption of dairy products, such as cheese and yogurt, in moderation

Mediterranean diet

1. Grilled tomato and eggplant stack:

1. Rounds cut from two medium eggplants
2. 2 large, sliced, ripe tomatoes
3. To taste, add salt and pepper.
4. Olive oil, 1/4 cup
5. freshly grated Parmesan cheese, 1/4 cup
6. Balsamic vinegar, two tablespoons
7. 2 teaspoons chopped fresh basil

Instructions:

1. Grill at a medium-high temperature.
2. Slices of eggplant and tomato are salted, peppered, and brushed with oil.
3. Slices of tomato and eggplant should be grilled for 3 to 4 minutes on each side, or until browned and soft.
4. Slices of tomato and eggplant should be placed on a serving tray after being removed from the grill.
5. The eggplant and tomato stacks should have the Parmesan cheese sprinkled on top of them.
6. Basil leaves should be cut and drizzled with balsamic vinegar.

2. Stuffed Peppers in the Greek Style:

1. 4 large, any color bell peppers
2. 1 pound of ground beef or lamb
3. 1 diced onion
4. 3 minced garlic cloves
5. 1 cup cooked rice, either white or brown
6. 1 diced tomato can
7. Salt and pepper, to taste. 1/4 cup chopped kalamata olives; 2 tablespoons chopped fresh parsley 2 tablespoons chopped fresh mint
8. 1 cup of feta cheese in crumbles

Instructions:

1. Turn on the 375°F oven.
2. Line a baking pan with parchment paper.
3. The bell peppers' tops should be cut off, and the seeds and membranes should be removed.
4. Put the peppers in the baking pan that has been prepared.
5. Cook the ground lamb or beef in a sizable skillet over medium heat, breaking it up into small pieces as it cooks.
6. When the onion is transparent, add it to the skillet along with the garlic.
7. Add the salt, pepper, parsley, mint, chopped tomatoes, and cooked rice after stirring.

8. Cook until well heated.

9. Fill the bell peppers evenly with the mixture by spoon.

10. The filled peppers should be covered with feta cheese crumbles.

11. Bake the dish with the foil on top for 30–35 minutes, or until the filling is hot and the peppers are soft.

3. Baked cod with lemon and herbs:

1. 4 filets of cod (6 ounces each)

2. To taste, add salt and pepper.

3. Olive oil, 1/4 cup

4. 2 lemons, cut 2 tablespoons of freshly chopped parsley 2 tablespoons freshly chopped basil 2 teaspoons of freshly chopped oregano

Instructions:

1. Set the oven to 400 °F. Use parchment paper to cover a baking sheet.

2. Olive oil should be brushed on after seasoning the cod filets with salt and pepper.

3. Place a couple lemon slices on top of each cod filet before placing it on the prepared baking sheet.

4. Top the cod filets with the chopped parsley, basil, and oregano.

5. Bake the fish for 12 to 15 minutes, or until it is thoroughly done and flaky.

4. Salad of chickpeas and feta:

1. 1 can of washed and drained chickpeas

2. One cucumber, chopped; half a red onion, thinly sliced; and one pint of cherry tomatoes.

3. 1/4 cup freshly cut parsley, 1/4 cup freshly chopped mint, and 1/4 cup freshly squeezed lemon juice

4. Olive oil, 3 tablespoons

5. Pepper and salt to taste 1

CHAPTER 2

Overview of ketogenic diet's

The ketogenic diet, commonly referred to as the "keto" diet, is a high-fat, low-carb diet that has been demonstrated to have a number of health advantages, including better insulin sensitivity and weight loss.

The goal of the ketogenic diet is to limit carbohydrate consumption to a level that causes the body to go into a state of ketosis, during which it uses fat for energy instead of glucose from carbohydrates.

It's critical to consume a lot of good fats, a modest quantity of protein, and very few carbohydrates when on a ketogenic diet.

A ketogenic diet often consists of the following foods:

- Poultry, fish, and meat
- Eggs Dairy items, including heavy cream, cheese, and butter
- Olive oil and other types of oils and fats
- Low-carb vegetables, including kale, broccoli, and spinach
- seeds and nuts

- Avocados
- Bread, pasta, sugar, and processed snacks are examples of high-carbohydrate items that should be avoided because they can cause you to exit ketosis very rapidly.

Advantages of ketogenic diet

The following are a few potential advantages of a ketogenic diet:

- ➤ Weight reduction: Since the body burns fat for energy, a diet heavy in fat and low in carbohydrates may cause rapid weight loss.
- ➤ Enhanced insulin sensitivity: The ketogenic diet can enhance insulin sensitivity and blood sugar control by reducing carbohydrate intake, which may be advantageous for people with type 2 diabetes.
    - → Energy levels rise when the body starts to burn fat for energy, according to many people who follow the ketogenic diet.

- ➤ improved brain function: The brain can use the ketones created during ketosis in place of the glucose it normally obtains from carbohydrates. This could result in enhanced cognitive function and fewer symptoms of neurodegenerative diseases.

→ While the ketogenic diet may offer a number of advantages, it can also be difficult to follow and may not be suitable for everyone. Before beginning any new diet, it is always advisable to see a healthcare professional, especially if you have any underlying medical issues.

1. Chicken breast wrapped in avocado and bacon

Ingredients:

1. Four skinless, boneless chicken breasts are the main component.
2. 8 bacon slices
3. Two mature avocados
4. To taste, add salt and pepper.
5. using olive oil to brush

Instructions:

1. Set the oven's temperature to 400°F (204°C).

2. Remove the pit from each avocado, cut it in half, and mash the flesh in a basin. To taste, add salt and pepper to the food.

3. On a chopping board, add a chicken breast and a teaspoon of the avocado mixture.

4. Two pieces of bacon should be wrapped around the outside of the chicken breast to secure it after rolling it up around the avocado mixture.

5. Use the remaining chicken breasts to repeat the process.

6. Olive oil should be used to brush on the chicken breasts before adding salt and pepper to taste.

7. The chicken breasts should be baked for 25 to 30 minutes, or until the bacon is crisp and the chicken is cooked through.

8. Serve warm alongside your preferred side dishes.

9. Fritters of zucchini with tzatziki sauce

2. Grated zucchini from two big zucchini

Ingredients:

1. all-purpose flour, 1/4 cup

2. 2 large, lightly beaten eggs

3. grated Parmesan cheese, 1/4 cup

4. To taste, add salt and pepper.

5. Use olive oil while cooking.

6. When making the tzatziki sauce:

7. 1 cup of unsweetened Greek yogurt

8. 12 cucumbers, grated after being peeled

9. 1 minced garlic clove

10. Lemon juice, one tablespoon

11. To taste, add salt and pepper.

Instructions:

1. Grated zucchini, flour, eggs, Parmesan cheese, salt, and pepper should all be combined in a large bowl.

2. Stir thoroughly to mix.

3. A big frying pan should be preheated over medium heat with just enough olive oil to cover the bottom.

4. Scoop up some of the zucchini mixture with a large spoon and drop it into the boiling oil. Use the back of the spoon to flatten the fritter.

5. Repeat the process with the remaining zucchini mixture, frying two to three fritters at once.

6. Fritters should be cooked for two to three minutes on each side, or until golden brown.

7. Take it out of the pan and let it dry on paper towels.

8. To prepare the tzatziki sauce, mix the grated cucumber, grated garlic, lemon juice, salt, and pepper in a small bowl with the Greek yogurt.

9. Stir thoroughly to mix.

10. With the Tzatziki Sauce on the side, serve the zucchini fritters hot.

3. Pork Chops with a Salad of Radish and Arugula

Ingredients:

1. 4 pork chops with bone
2. To taste, add salt and pepper.
3. using olive oil to brush

To make the salad:

1. Arugula, 4 cups
2. 8 sliced thin radishes
3. 1/4 cup of goat cheese crumbles
4. Lemon juice, one tablespoon
5. To taste, add salt and pepper.

Instructions:

1. Set the oven's temperature to 400°F (204°C).
2. Add salt and pepper to taste and season the pork chops.

3. a big oven-safe skillet over medium heat.

Overview of smoothies and juicing

Two well-liked techniques for including more fruits and veggies in your diet are juicing and smoothies. Both have advantages of their own, and lots of individuals combine the two in their diets.

Juicing is the process of removing the juice alone from fruits and vegetables, leaving the fiber behind. As a result, the body receives a concentrated amount of vitamins, minerals, and antioxidants. For those who struggle to eat enough fruits and vegetables, juicing might be a handy approach to increasing their intake. Juicing can, however, be very rich in sugar, so it's advised to reduce the amount of sweet fruit juices and increase the number of green vegetables in the juice.

On the other hand, complete fruits and vegetables—including the fiber—are blended in smoothies. This offers a source of nutrients that is more evenly distributed, including fiber, which helps to control blood sugar levels and encourage feelings of fullness.

Smoothies can be a great way to increase the amount of fruits and vegetables in your diet, but it's important to remember that they can also be high in sugar and calories. To balance the sugar in your smoothies, add protein and healthy fats.

Both juicing and smoothies have potential health advantages, such as improving digestion, boosting immunity, lowering inflammation, and fostering general health and wellness.

However, it's crucial to keep in mind that they are to be used as a supplement to a balanced diet rather than as the only source of

Smoothies and juicing

Green Detox Juice: Berries and Spinach Smoothie Immune-Boosting Citrus Smoothie Carrot-Ginger Juice

1. Green Detox Juice:

Ingredients:

1. Kale, two hefty handfuls
2. 1-inch cucumber
3. 2 apples of medium size
4. One medium lemon
5. piece of ginger, 1 inch long.

Instructions:

1. All ingredients should be clean and ready.
2. Apply a juicer to the kale, cucumber, apples, lemon, and ginger.

2. Ginger-Carrot Juice: Components:

1. four medium carrots
2. a single medium apple
3. piece of ginger, 1 inch long.

Instructions:

1. All ingredients should be clean and ready.
2. Use a juicer to process the carrots, apple, and ginger.

3. Smoothie with spinach and berries:

1. one cup of mixed frozen berries
2. one cup of spinach
3. one banana
4. Almond milk, half a cup
5. 1 scoop of protein powder in vanilla (optional)

Instructions:

1. All ingredients should be clean and ready.
2. Blend all ingredients in a blender until they are completely smooth.

4. Smoothie with citrus to strengthen the immune system:

1. one medium grapefruit
2. One medium orange
3. one banana
4. frozen strawberries, half a cup
5. Coconut water, 1/2 cup

Instructions:

1. All ingredients should be clean and ready.
2. Blend all ingredients in a blender until they are completely smooth.

Serve it right away and delight in it!

Overview of Gerson therapy diet

Gerson Therapy is a nutritional strategy that is predicated on the idea that consuming full, organic, and fresh foods can promote the body's innate capacity to heal itself of chronic and degenerative illnesses, including cancer.

The following tenets underpin the therapy, according to the Gerson Institute:

consuming a lot of organic fruits and vegetables to acquire the necessary enzymes, antioxidants, and nutrients.

A rich amount of nutrients can be obtained by consuming raw juices produced from organic fruits and vegetables multiple times per day.

avoiding harmful fats, refined sugars, and processed foods.

eating a vegetarian, low-sodium diet.

bodily cleansing with the aid of coffee enemas and vitamins.

There is little scientific evidence to support the usefulness of the Gerson therapy as a standard cancer treatment, and it is not usually acknowledged as such. Additionally, some of the therapy's components, such as coffee enemas, might be harmful and need to only be carried out under a doctor's supervision.

It's crucial to remember that each person has unique health requirements, and what works for one person might not work for another. Before changing your diet or treatment regimen, it is always advisable to speak with a trained healthcare practitioner, especially when it comes to serious medical illnesses like cancer.

1. Juice from fresh vegetables

Ingredients:

1. 4 big carrots
2. 2 apples of medium size
3. a single little beet
4. one medium cucumber
5. 2 substantial handfuls of spinach

Instructions:

1. All ingredients should be clean and ready.
2. Juice the spinach, apples, beets, cucumbers, and carrots.

2. Soup with lentils and vegetables

Ingredients:

1. 1 cup of rinsed and drained green lentils
2. 1 big, chopped onion
3. 2 minced garlic cloves
4. 2 chopped medium-sized carrots
5. two medium-sized celery stalks, chopped
6. 1 chopped medium-sized zucchini
7. 4 cups of veggie stock
8. one tomato chopped in a can

9. Olive oil, 2 tablespoons

10. pepper and salt as desired.

Instructions:

1. In a sizable saucepan set over medium heat, warm the olive oil.

2. About 5 minutes after adding them, the onion and garlic should be tender and fragrant.

3. For a further five minutes, add the zucchini, celery, and carrots and continue to sauté.

4. Bring to a boil the lentils, vegetable broth, diced tomatoes, salt, and pepper in a saucepan.

5. Once the lentils are tender, lower the heat and let the soup simmer for around 30 minutes.

3. Sweet potatoes baked with almond butter

Ingredients:

1. Two little sweet potatoes

2. Almond butter, two tablespoons

3. Salt as desired.

Instructions:

1. Set the oven to 400°F.

2. The sweet potatoes should be washed, dried, and forked numerous times.

3. Bake the sweet potatoes for 45 to 50 minutes, or until they are tender and soft, on a baking sheet.

4. Give the sweet potatoes some time to cool.

5. Each sweet potato should be split lengthwise, and the centers of each half should each contain a spoonful of almond butter.

4. Pesto-topped cauliflower rice with cherry tomatoes:

Ingredients:

1. 1 cauliflower head, cut into florets

2. pesto of basil, half a cup

3. 1 cup of halved cherry tomatoes

4. pepper and salt as desired.

Instructions:

1. When the cauliflower is reduced to rice-sized bits, add the cauliflower florets to a food processor and pulse a few times.

2. The cauliflower rice should be heated in a sizable saucepan over medium heat for about 5 minutes, or until it is cooked through and slightly browned.

3. Heat for an additional two to three minutes, or
    until the cherry tomatoes are heated through,
    then stir in the pesto.

CHAPTER 3

Overview of Macrobiotic diet

The macrobiotic diet is an all-encompassing way of eating that places an emphasis on whole, unprocessed, and natural foods.

It is based on the Yin and Yang theory, which holds that all substances and actions may be divided into two categories: Yin (cool, passive, and yielding) and Yang (hot, active, and aggressive).

To maintain general health and ward off sickness, the macrobiotic diet tries to achieve balance between yin and yang foods in the diet.

The following are a few of the main advantages of the macrobiotic diet:

Promotes Whole Foods: The macrobiotic diet places a strong emphasis on natural, unprocessed foods that are free of additives and chemicals, which can help lower the chance of developing chronic diseases like diabetes, heart disease, and cancer.

Hormone Balance: The macrobiotic diet places a strong emphasis on consuming plant-based foods that are full of phytoestrogens, which can help regulate hormones and lower the risk of hormonal abnormalities.

Supports Digestion: The macrobiotic diet includes fermented foods, which are high in probiotics and can support digestive health and ward off ailments like irritable bowel syndrome (IBS) and bloating. These foods include miso, pickles, and tempeh.

Reduces Inflammation: The macrobiotic diet is full of anti-inflammatory foods, including whole grains, veggies, and legumes, which can lower your risk of developing chronic illnesses like rheumatoid arthritis and osteoporosis.

Promotes Sustainability: The macrobiotic diet places a strong emphasis on locally grown, seasonally available, and organic foods, which can assist in lowering carbon emissions and advancing sustainability.

Brown rice, whole grain bread, miso soup, sea vegetables, fermented foods, legumes, and seasonal fruits and vegetables are a few examples of items that are frequently eaten on the macrobiotic diet.

Some recipes that are suitable for macrobiotics are:
- A recipe for miso soup with tofu and wakame is given below:

Ingredients:
1. 4 cups of liquid
2. Two teaspoons of wakame seaweed, dried
3. Miso paste, 4 teaspoons
4. Cubed tofu in a half-cup
5. 2 sliced green onions
6. toasted sesame oil, 1 teaspoon

Instructions:
1. Bring the water to a boil in a big pot.
2. Ten minutes later, add the wakame seaweed and let it soak.
3. Take out and set aside the wakame seaweed.
4. To make a smooth paste, combine the miso paste and a tiny amount of the hot water in a small bowl.
5. Stir well after adding the miso paste to the pot with the remaining hot water.
6. Let the soup simmer for two to three minutes after adding the tofu and green onions.

7. Add the wakame seaweed after taking the soup off the heat.

8. Serve hot with the sesame oil drizzled over top.

- A recipe for a brown rice and vegetable bowl is provided below.

Ingredients:

1. 1 serving of brown rice
2. 2 glasses of water
3. Sea salt, 1 teaspoon
4. 12 cups of diced carrots
5. chopped bell peppers, 1/2 cup
6. Zucchini, chopped into half a cup
7. 1/2 cup of yellow squash dice
8. Olive oil, 2 tablespoons
9. Tamari, two tablespoons
10. Juice of two teaspoons of lemon
11. Sesame seeds, roasted, in 2 teaspoons

Instructions:

1. Drain the brown rice after giving it a cold-water rinse.
2. Bring the water and sea salt to a boil in a saucepan.
3. Brown rice should be added before the pan is covered.

4. For 40 minutes, turn the heat down to low and cook the rice.

5. Olive oil should be heated in a sizable skillet over medium heat.

6. Stir-fry the vegetables for 5–7 minutes after adding the carrots, bell peppers, zucchini, and yellow squash.

7. To prepare the dressing, combine the tamari, lemon juice, and toasted sesame seeds in a small bowl.

8. Place the stir-fried vegetables on top of the brown rice when serving it in a bowl.

9. Serve after drizzling the dressing over top.

- Here is a recipe for a stir-fry with seitan and vegetables:

Ingredients:

1. Seitan, 1 packet

2. Cornstarch, two teaspoons

3. Olive oil, 2 tablespoons

4. diced onions, half a cup

5. 12 cups of diced carrots

6. chopped bell peppers, 1/2 cup

7. Zucchini, chopped into half a cup

8. Tamari, two tablespoons

9. Honey, 1 tablespoon

10. Rice vinegar, 1 tbsp.

11. toasted sesame oil, 1 teaspoon

Instructions:

1. Sprinkle it with cornstarch after slicing the seitan into thin pieces.

2. Olive oil should be heated in a sizable skillet over medium heat.

3. Stir-fry the seitan for 5–7 minutes, or until golden brown.

4. From the skillet, take out and reserve the seitan.

5. Add the onions, carrots, bell peppers, and zucchini to the same skillet and stir-fry for 5 to 7 minutes.

6. To prepare the sauce, combine the tamari, honey, rice vinegar, and toasted sesame oil in a small bowl.

7. Re-add the seitan to the pan

Overview of alkaline diet

The idea behind the alkaline diet, often referred to as the "alkaline ash diet," is that particular foods can change the pH balance of the body and encourage an alkaline environment.

An alkaline environment, according to proponents of this diet, can help lower the risk of chronic illnesses like cancer and enhance general health.

While avoiding processed and acidic foods like meat, dairy, and sugar, the alkaline diet emphasizes the consumption of whole, plant-based foods, including fruits, vegetables, whole grains, legumes, and nuts.

- The following are a few of the alleged advantages of an alkaline diet:

Improved digestion: Eating a diet high in foods that promote alkalinity can aid digestion and lessen acid reflux symptoms.

Immune system stimulation: Consuming alkaline foods can aid in enhancing immunity and reducing inflammation.

pH balance maintained: The alkaline diet can help lower the risk of chronic diseases and enhance general health by maintaining the pH levels in the body.

Increased energy: The alkaline diet can aid in boosting energy levels and enhancing athletic performance by lowering the body's acid load.

Better bone health: By lowering the risk of osteoporosis and boosting bone density, an alkaline diet may promote bone health.

Even though there is some scientific proof that an alkaline diet can improve health, it is crucial to remember that more research is required to completely grasp both its potential advantages and disadvantages.

As with any diet, it is imperative to speak with a healthcare provider before making any changes to your eating habits.

Alkaline diet

- Grapefruit and avocado salad:

Ingredients:

1. 2 diced ripe avocados

2. 2 segmented and peeled grapefruits
3. freshly squeezed lemon juice, 2 tablespoons
4. Olive oil, extra virgin, two tablespoons
5. To taste, add salt and black pepper.
6. Uncountable mixed greens

Instructions:

1. Mix the diced avocado and grapefruit segments carefully in a large bowl.
2. Combine the lemon juice, olive oil, salt, and pepper in a small bowl.
3. After adding the dressing, gently toss the avocado and grapefruit combination together.
4. On top of a bed of mixed greens, plate the salad.

- Bell peppers stuffed with quinoa and vegetables

Ingredients:

1. 4 large bell peppers, seeded and cut in half.
2. 1 cup cooked quinoa
3. 1 cup of various vegetables (such as diced carrots, zucchini, and mushrooms)
4. 1 can of washed and drained chickpeas
5. 1/9 cup cumin
6. To taste, add salt and black pepper.
7. tomato sauce, 1 cup

Instructions:

1. Turn the oven on to 375°F.
2. Combine the cooked quinoa, mixed vegetables, chickpeas, cumin, salt, and pepper in a sizable bowl.
3. The quinoa mixture should be placed inside each bell pepper half.
4. In a baking dish, put the filled bell peppers and top with tomato sauce.
5. Bake the bell peppers for 25 to 30 minutes, or until they are soft and the filling is hot.

- Green Alkaline Smoothie:

Ingredients:

1. one banana
2. spinach, 1 cup
3. almond milk, 1 cup
4. Chia seeds, one tablespoon
5. 1 tsp. of honey
6. one-half teaspoon of vanilla extract

Instructions:

1. Banana, spinach, almond milk, chia seeds, honey, and vanilla essence should all be put in a blender.
2. Blend until smooth on high.

3. Pour into a glass, then sip.

- Skewers of grilled tofu and vegetables:

Ingredients:
1. 1 block of firm tofu, cut into cubes after being drained
2. two bell peppers, seeded, and diced
3. a single big onion, diced
4. sliced zucchini from 2
5. Olive oil, two tablespoons
6. To taste, add salt and black pepper.
7. 8 wooden skewers soaked for 30 minutes in water

Instructions:
1. Combine the tofu, bell peppers, onions, and zucchini in a sizable bowl.
2. Sprinkle it with salt and pepper and drizzle with olive oil.
3. The soaking skewers are then threaded with the vegetables and tofu.
4. The grill or grill pan should be heated to medium-high.
5. Turn them every few minutes, grill the skewers for 10–15 minutes, or until the tofu is gently browned and the vegetables are soft.

Overview of fasting diets

Dietary patterns known as fasting diets feature intervals of little or no food consumption. Due to the potential health advantages of this diet, such as possible weight loss, increased insulin sensitivity, and decreased inflammation, it has become more and more popular in recent years.

Fasting diets come in a variety of forms, each with a special strategy. Popular fasting diets consist of:

Intermittent Fasting: This entails alternating between eating and fasting for short windows of time, usually between 16 and 24 hours.

Alternate-Day Fasting: This involves switching back and forth between days when you eat normally and days when you don't.

Time-Restricted Feeding: This entails limiting the time of day during which you eat, usually between six and twelve hours.

Prolonged fasting: This involves going without food for a lengthy time, usually 2–7 days.

Studies have revealed that fasting diets can improve a number of health indicators, such as lowering the risk of chronic diseases, enhancing cognitive function, and extending life.

Fasting diets, however, should only be followed with the advice of a healthcare provider because they can be difficult and even harmful for some people, such as those with a history of disordered eating or medical issues.

- Cold soup with cucumber and mint:

Ingredients:

1. Cucumbers, 4 medium, peeled and chopped
2. two cups of vegetable stock
3. Greek yogurt, plain, in 1/2 cup
4. Fresh mint leaves, 1/4 cup
5. one garlic clove
6. 1 teaspoon of lemon juice
7. pepper and salt as desired.

Instructions:

Cucumbers that have been cut, Greek yogurt, mint leaves, garlic, and lemon juice should all be combined in a blender.

Until smooth, blend.

To taste, add salt and pepper to the food.

Before serving, let the food cool in the refrigerator for at least two hours.

- Salad of spinach and fennel:

Ingredients:

1. 4 cups fresh leaves of spinach
2. 1 large, finely sliced fennel bulb
3. thinly slice 1 medium red onion
4. 14 cups lightly toasted almonds
5. 1/4 cup feta cheese crumbles
6. 2/TBSP of olive oil
7. Balsamic vinegar, 1 tablespoon
8. pepper and salt as desired.

Instructions:

1. The spinach leaves, fennel slices, red onion, toasted almonds, and feta cheese should all be combined in a big bowl.
2. Combine the olive oil and balsamic vinegar in a small bowl.

3. After adding the dressing, toss the salad to incorporate it.
4. To taste, add salt and pepper to the food.

- Carrot and sweet potato soup:

Ingredients:
1. Chop two medium sweet potatoes after peeling them.
2. Cut four medium carrots after peeling them.
3. two cups of vegetable stock
4. Dry thyme, 1 teaspoon
5. 1 teaspoon cumin
6. pepper and salt as desired.

Instructions:
1. Sweet potatoes, carrots, thyme, cumin, and vegetable broth all go into a big saucepan.
2. Bring to a boil, then lower the heat and simmer for 20 to 25 minutes, or until the veggies are fork-tender.

3. The soup should be pureed until smooth using an immersion blender or by transferring to a blender.
4. To taste, add salt and pepper to the food.

- Chickpea Salad with Herbs:

Ingredients:

1. 1 can of washed and drained chickpeas
2. 1 chopped medium red bell pepper
3. diced one medium cucumber.
4. 14 cups finely minced fresh parsley
5. 14 cups finely minced fresh basil
6. 1 teaspoon lemon juice
7. 2/TBSP of olive oil
8. pepper and salt as desired.

Instructions:

1. Chickpeas, chopped bell pepper, cucumber, parsley, and basil should all be combined in a big basin.
2. Combine the lemon juice and olive oil in a small bowl.
3. After adding the dressing, toss the salad to incorporate it.
4. To taste, add salt and pepper to the food.

BONUS PAGE

List of desserts that combat cancer

When thinking about a diet to prevent cancer, dessert may not necessarily be the first thing that springs to mind, but it is still feasible to indulge in a sweet treat while promoting your general health.

Here is a list of desserts that combat cancer:

Fruit that is still in season is the best method to satisfy your sweet tooth while also getting the necessary vitamins and minerals. Particularly berries, which are strong in antioxidants and have been demonstrated to have anti-cancer effects.

Dark Chocolate: Flavonoids, a class of chemicals with demonstrated anti-cancer potential, are abundant in dark chocolate. To reap the greatest health benefits, choose dark chocolate that contains a high amount of cocoa solids.

Desserts made using sweet potatoes: sweet potatoes are rich in anti-inflammatory and antioxidant components. For a tasty and nutritious dessert, try sweet potato pie, sweet potato muffins, or sweet potato cake.

Desserts made with almond milk: For those looking for a diet that fights cancer, almond milk is a perfect substitute for dairy. Almonds alone contain a lot of anti-inflammatory and antioxidant chemicals. For a tasty and nutritious treat, try making almond milk ice cream, pudding, or smoothies.

Desserts made with green tea: Green tea contains a lot of catechins, which have been demonstrated to have anti-cancer qualities. For a tasty and nutritious treat, try preparing green tea ice cream, green tea cake, or green tea cookies.

Even when eating dessert, it's still crucial to keep your intake of sugar and processed foods to a minimum. The key is moderation, and choosing healthier foods when you can can assist you in keeping up a healthy, cancer-fighting diet.

- Salad with fresh fruit, lime, and mint:

Ingredients:

1. 2 cups of fresh fruit mixture (such as berries, melon, and sliced grapes)
2. 2 tablespoons of finely chopped fresh mint leaves

3. freshly squeezed lime juice, 2 tablespoons

4. 1 teaspoon of honey (optional)

Instructions:

Fruit should be washed and diced into bite-sized pieces.

Combine the fruit, mint leaves, lime juice, and honey in a large basin (if using).

Gently blend by tossing.

Serve right away or chill in the fridge until you're ready to.

- Apples baked with walnuts and cinnamon:

Ingredients:

1. Four big apples

2. 14 cups chopped walnuts

3. Brown sugar, 2 tablespoons

4. 1 cinnamon stick

5. 1/8 nutmeg teaspoon

6. 2 teaspoons of tiny chunks of unsalted butter

Instructions:

1. Set the oven's temperature to 375°F (190°C).

2. Apples should be cored and sliced thin.

3. Combine the walnuts, brown sugar, cinnamon, and nutmeg in a sizable bowl.

4. Put the apple slices in a 9-inch (23-cm) baking dish in a single layer.

5. The walnut mixture should be strewn over the apples.

6. Sprinkle the butter chunks on top.

7. Bake the dish for 15 minutes while it is covered with aluminum foil.

8. When the apples are soft and the topping is crispy, remove the foil and bake for an additional 15 minutes.

- Fruit and Chia Seed Pudding:

Ingredients:

1. 1 cup of almond milk without sugar

2. Chia seeds, 1/4 cup

3. Vanilla extract, 1 teaspoon

4. 1 teaspoon of honey

5. 1 cup of fresh berries blended (such as strawberries, blueberries, and raspberries)

Instructions:

1. Mix the almond milk, chia seeds, honey, vanilla, and extract in a big basin.

2. Overnight or for at least two hours, cover and chill.

3. Prior to serving, stir the ingredients.

4. Place the mixed berries on top of the pudding after dividing it into individual serving bowls.

- Banana Bread Without Gluten:

Ingredients:

1. 1 1/2 cups all-purpose gluten-free flour
2. one tablespoon of baking powder
3. A half-teaspoon of baking soda
4. 0.5 teaspoons of salt
5. 12 cups softened unsalted butter
6. One sugar cup
7. two huge eggs
8. Vanilla extract, 1 teaspoon
9. ripe bananas mashed to 1 1/2 cups (about 3 medium)
10. chopped walnuts, half a cup (optional)

Instructions:

1. Set the oven's temperature to 350°F (180°C).
2. A 9x5-inch (23x13cm) loaf pan should be greased.
3. Mix the flour, baking soda, baking powder, and salt in a medium bowl.
4. Cream the butter and sugar in a sizable basin until they are light and creamy.
5. One at a time, beat in the eggs. Next, add the vanilla extract and mashed bananas.

6. Mix just till mixed after gradually incorporating the dry ingredients into the wet ones.

7. If using, stir in the chopped walnuts.

8. Put the prepared loaf pan with the batter inside.

9. A toothpick inserted in the center of the cake should come out clean after baking for 60 to 70 minutes

10. 10 minutes should pass while the bread cools in the pan.

Final thoughts on the significance of a diet that fights cancer.

Overview of the Main Takeaways

Understanding the Relationship Between Diet and Cancer: Our diet can significantly affect both our chance of having cancer and our capacity to treat and recover from it.

Diets based on plants: Diets based on plants are full of vitamins, minerals, fiber, and antioxidants that can prevent cancer and enhance general health.

Diets that are anti-inflammatory: Diets that are anti-inflammatory can assist to lessen chronic inflammation in the body, which is a major factor in the development of cancer.

The Mediterranean diet places a strong emphasis on complete, unprocessed foods like fruits, vegetables, whole grains, and healthy fats, which can help lower the risk of cancer and enhance general health.

The ketogenic diet is a low-carb, high-fat diet that can prevent cancer by boosting ketone synthesis and lowering blood glucose levels.

Smoothies and juices: Smoothies and juices can give the body a concentrated amount of antioxidants, vitamins, and minerals that can help fight cancer.

The Gerson Therapy Diet is a plant-based eating plan that places a focus on fresh, organic fruits and vegetables, which can promote the body's natural healing processes.

The macrobiotic diet is a plant-based diet centered on the concepts of harmony and balance that emphasizes whole, unprocessed foods such grains, legumes, and vegetables.

The alkaline diet focuses on eating things that keep the body's pH levels in a healthy range, which can help lower the risk of cancer and enhance general health.

Fasting Diets: Oxidative stress, a major factor in the development of cancer, can be lessened and the body can detoxify with the use of fasting diets.

Choices for desserts that fight cancer Desserts that are delicious and healthful, including fresh fruit salad, baked apples, and chia seed pudding, can give the body a boost of minerals and antioxidants that fight cancer.

Final Reflections: An essential part of comprehensive cancer care and prevention is a cancer-fighting diet. We may help our bodies fight cancer naturally by including full, unprocessed foods like fruits, vegetables, whole grains, and healthy fats in our diets.

Include foods that are known to be effective in the battle against cancer, such as those included in plant-based, anti-inflammatory, and alkaline diets.

A healthcare professional should be consulted before making any significant dietary modifications.